SIXTY... so what?

SIXTY... so what?

A Handbook for
Staying Young
at Sixty

SHARON JONES, Ph.D

Tate Publishing & *Enterprises*

Sixty...So What?

This title is also available as a Tate Out Loud product. Visit www.tatepublishing.com for more information.

Published by Tate Publishing & Enterprises, LLC
127 E. Trade Center Terrace | Mustang, Oklahoma 73064 USA
1.888.361.9473 | www.tatepublishing.com

Tate Publishing is committed to excellence in the publishing industry. The company reflects the philosophy established by the founders, based on Psalms 68:11,
"The Lord gave the word and great was the company of those who published it."

Cover design by Taylor Rauschkolb
Interior design by Leah LeFlore
Cover photo by Lonnie Kees of Lonnie Kees Photography, Jackson, MS.
Published in the United States of America

ISBN: 978-1-60247-465-9

07.05.14

Table of Contents

Introduction

Okay, let's face it, you wouldn't be reading this book if you weren't close to that "age." You may be in your late fifties and are dreading the years that our youth-oriented society has termed "senior." Well, I have good news for you. There is a positive change on the horizon, and you can be a part of that revolution. Our generation has embraced a different attitude toward aging than our parent's generation. Don't you remember that when you were forty, you considered a sixty-year-old woman "old"? Well, no more. Sixty-year-old women are embracing new challenges, which may include a return to college for a Ph.D., or simply letting their hair grow longer than once thought fashionable. We no longer have to wear sensible shoes that protect our feet. We have pedicures and wear the sandals our daughters are emoting over. If, by chance, we fall, we'll look good as we land!

So, you are wondering by now how I became qualified to write this book that I hope will become an invaluable tool as you embark upon this aging process. My first qualification is my birth date of June 13, 1944. My second and probably the most important qualification is that on June 8, 2005, I became Dr. Jones. Sounds good, doesn't it? You do the math. I was sixty. You can do it; you can achieve whatever you desire. This handbook is your guide to aging with grace and style. You will understand how reaching the years that you may have dreaded can be the very best of your life. Now, let's see how you can make that happen.

Why Does My Attitude Matter?

Your attitude has always been a factor in your mental and spiritual growth. You can choose to be happy or unhappy. You can choose to be the best you can be, or just give up and blame your age. Sadly, many women have done just that. You see them everyday... women who have given up. *You do not have to be that woman.* That's not fair to you or your family. Your age should never become a factor in your attitude. So what do you do? You find your passion. No, I don't mean sex. What, at your age? (Of course, at your age, but I will save that for another book.)

How do you capture that passion? One avenue is to pretend that you are thirty again. What would you do? Make a list of your interests. Since age is not a factor in this equation, you can dream of anything. Did you want to become a lawyer when you were younger and before life got in the way? Well, it doesn't have to now. Make the first step and send for a graduate bulletin of the law school closest to you. Just the bulletin; you are not ready for the LSAT (the test you must take to enter law school). I'm sure you get the point. You have to make a step in the direction of your dream. Maybe your dream is just to finish your degree. Call the college or university near you. There has been an influx during the last decade of non-traditional students (as you would be) on our college campuses. How do I know that? I am a sociology professor who received a Ph.D. at the age of sixty. I was the oldest student in my class and one of the first in my cohort to finish the requirements for the terminal degree. I was very proud. This can happen to you. My story is an example of a passion that became a reality.

Your passion may take a different approach. Remember, it is your passion. It belongs to no one but you. You may want to become a poet or a dancer. You may want to be a designer or an artist. You must find your passion; focus on this passion, and it will become your reality. What are you waiting for? The reality is that you deserve to pursue this dream. You must start today by doing something that will lead you in that direction. If you do it now, you will have many years to enjoy your labor.

This is your workbook. No one has to see it unless you choose to share your dreams with them. Now let's get started. I want you to list five steps that you will take to make your passion a reality. For example, when I decided to return to school, I took an English course at a local community college. I loved it. I stopped only one semester to marry the man of my dreams, who became my most ardent cheerleader. Tragically, he died in an accident before I received my undergraduate degree. Knowing what it would have meant to him, I completed my undergraduate work after his death and then went on to obtain my master's degree. I thought it was enough, but it wasn't. I waited five years before I returned to work on my Ph.D. I would have never been satisfied if I had not tried. I am sure you will feel the same. You must get started today. Do something to reach your goal. Just making this important list below is your first step. You are on your way!

Now list your five steps before we go on to the next chapter:

1. ____

2. ____

3. ____

4. ____

5. ____

Why Are My Relationships Important?

Relationships cover a myriad of the people who are in your life. You may have been married for many years, and if you have had the good sense to have stayed married to your best friend, then you are indeed a very fortunate woman. Not all of us are so privileged. Many of us find ourselves in bad marriages. Many of us have experienced a late-life divorce and must find the courage to start over and forge a new life for ourselves. Many of us are widows who haven't learned how to be on our own without a man to define and protect us.

I am not a psychologist and cannot give you professional advice on the relationships that you may have or wish you could have with a man. I can, however, give you some important and practical advice on the relationships that you should have with a group of female friends. I hope that you can name at least four or five girlfriends whom you would like to have with you on a fun "girl's weekend." I have that! I can't tell you how important it is to have traveling buddies. If you haven't had that experience, what are you waiting for? If you have a husband, encourage him to promote your weekend with the girls, and I promise you he will have a wife with a different attitude when you return. If you don't have a husband, I really don't understand why you haven't been on a girl's trip. Start making your plans now!

Another important relationship that you might have overlooked is the possibility of adopting a pet. This can add a very important dimension to your life, especially if you are alone. My husband died in January of 1995, and after ten months of being alone, I decided to add a little fluff-puff of a dog to my household. I named her Shachet Elizabeth Jones, and she became my baby. I was possessed. I bought her clothes, furniture, and insurance. I took her to the vet if she sneezed and called him her "pediatrician." She lived for ten years and brought much joy to all who knew her. If you are lonely, I highly recommend a pet for company. You do realize a pet will give you unconditional love, never talk back, and will never try to trade you in on a younger model. Enough said?

The focus of this chapter has been to explore the possibilities of your relationships. The most important relationship you can have is with yourself. Yes, with you. You must learn to respect, like, and even love being with "you" before you can enjoy being with anyone else. Either you have a busy family life, a husband, a roommate, or you live alone. The circumstances aren't relevant. You must learn to enjoy your own company. Statistics tell us that 80% of married women today will be widowed. These are staggering statistics, which, compiled with the divorce statistics, point to a very strong possibility that you will spend some of your future years alone. Therefore, you must learn to be your own best friend. I realize that is hard to do. Again, start with small changes. Think of one thing that you would like to do for yourself. Think of something that you enjoy. It can be buying a new magazine on a subject that you are interested in and taking time to carefully peruse its pages. It can be taking a trip to the mall with nothing in mind to buy, but taking your time looking in a store you haven't been in before. If you can't bring yourself to have lunch in a restaurant alone, then you might have a sandwich in the food court at the mall. Start with these small steps, and you will find out that you just may enjoy being alone with your new friend . . . you.

Your assignment in this chapter is to list five activities that you might enjoy doing alone. You won't really be alone since you are developing this new friendship with you!

Now list these activities. It doesn't matter what they are since this is your workbook and no one else will have access to your thoughts unless you share. I know you are wondering why I am always asking you to list certain ideas. It is important to see your thoughts on paper. It makes your actions much easier to accomplish.

So, make your list and have fun!

1. ____

2. ____

3. ____

4. ____

5. ____

Why Can't I Lose Weight?

I wish I had an accurate count of all the diet and exercise books I have purchased in the past twenty years. They were each destined to make me exactly the weight I wanted to be by just reading them. Of course, you know that is a fallacy. I know you are waiting for me to tell you that I had a weight problem and that I uncovered some hidden weight loss secret. I wish I could. I have never been over ten pounds above my desired weight, but I have lost and gained those ten pounds many, many times. When I do reach my weight goal after much dieting and deprivation (or so it seems), I become careless and feel that I deserve to be enjoying whatever delectable dish I can obtain. Well, you know the drill. First, one pound, and then three, and soon the ten pounds are back. I panic and start the process over. I do my research and select the newest diet to throw myself into. It doesn't work!

I will share with you what has worked for me. This has been an almost recent discovery. I decided to quit dieting. I know you have heard that also. Well, it has worked for me. Actually, I have devised an eating plan that has worked for me. I do try to avoid the "white" stuff and the "sweet" stuff. I know what you are thinking... *What fun is that?* A typical day for me would be wheat toast with a very good fat free spray butter and coffee for breakfast. For lunch I might have a salad with grilled chicken and a fat free raspberry dressing. For dinner I might sauté an onion in olive oil and add a chicken breast to simmer until it is done. Try it, it's great. With a fresh tomato or a similar addition, dinner is served. I know, it is more difficult when you have a family or a man to consider. Just add more chicken. Why shouldn't he be healthy also?

Remember the first chapter about attitude; well, your attitude is very important, as you already know. Say this to yourself, *I may be sixty or close to it, and I can't control that, but I can control my weight and my physical well-being*. We have all been in the mall or somewhere similar and have seen a woman who appears to be our age, but she looks to us like a movie star. All we want to do is crawl home and throw away the outfit we are wearing. We have to blame something outside ourselves. It may be ten pounds standing between you and that "look" from someone else. Let me add here, it is not all about looks; health is an important factor. A ten-pound weight loss can be a great health benefit. Just ask your doctor.

Okay, let's get back to looks. I did the health benefit insert because I do believe it, but I believe that most of you want to hear me discuss the reason you bought the book, which is so you can say, "Sixty... So What?" So, to be able to make that statement, you must be at a weight that looks good on you. You must adjust your attitude to compensate for all the fun lunches and romantic dinners that you will have in your future. You know what I mean. You are meeting your girlfriends at a new "ladies spot," and you want to try some of the delectable desserts. Try them, but have only a few bites. You can do it. Attitude, remember. Look at these outings as a challenge. You can have fun, yet stay on your personal eating plan. Watch the small things. In the south, sweet tea is the house wine. You don't need sweet tea. You don't need to drink your calories. Find a system that works for you.

This chapter is supposed to answer your question as to why you can't lose weight. I can only answer for myself... I eat too much. Does that sound familiar? So, I am not suggesting a diet. You must find your own eating plan. You are a smart woman. I am suggesting a change in attitude. You must believe that you can be the best you have ever been. Now this is not going to be accomplished in a short period of time. This change in your eating habits must be a permanent change. You must be ready to do this.

I am going to give you some pointers that have helped me reach my goal. I am almost there. You must not let yourself get hungry. You will not starve yourself into a smaller dress size. You will break down and have a binge of all the foods you have been craving. Make it a game and find the foods that satisfy you for a limited number of calories and fat grams. Fresh fruits have helped me satisfy the craving for something sweet, while pickled okra (yes, you can find it in the grocery store) has satisfied my craving for salty. And, it is true, you should drink water. Women with beautiful bodies seem to have a water bottle with them. Try it. Another secret, I really am telling you all of my secrets, is to take two fiber capsules and drink a glass of water before meals. The fiber is good for you, and I have found that it takes the edge off my hunger.

The most important part of a weight-loss program is to decide to do it and let nothing stop you. You will be proud as you shop for clothing in your new size, or if you are like I am, just look in your closet.

Now let's get started. You know I want you to list your goals and your steps to reach these weight loss goals. You can do it. I believe in you!

Now list them:

1. ______________________________

2. ______________________________

3. ______________________________

4. ______________________________

5. ______________________________

Why Do I Have to Exercise?

This will be the shortest chapter in the book. I don't like to exercise. I say that I do. I try to believe that I do, but I will put if off if I can get by with it. Well, you and I have to face the well-documented fact that exercise is the "fountain of youth." If we change the word exercise to activity, could you handle it better? Well, let's see. You need to be active everyday! You have read all the books and magazines that encourage you to park away from the front door of the mall and walk those extra steps; well, I confess that I don't do it, and I don't imagine that you do it either.

So, what can you do? I will tell you what I do, and you might glean something that will work for you. I have always tried to walk on a rather consistent basis. I am not a race walker, but a walker who thinks a mile around the neighborhood is sufficient. I know I could do more, but it never seems to happen. I live in Mississippi, and the summers are very hot and humid, therefore walking outside is not always an option. I will tell you what my back-up exercise is, and you may want to try it. I trampoline. I use a mini-trampoline that I bought many years ago for less than thirty dollars. I don't know what they cost now, but I am sure they are still an exercise equipment bargain. Therefore, if you will jog for ten to thirty minutes daily on this exercise equipment bargain, you will see some amazing results. Now, don't tell me you can't devote a certain amount of time to your new and easy exercise program daily. Attitude, remember?

If you are a seasoned exerciser you don't need this chapter, but if you are like the rest of us, you need to make an effort to add some exercise (activity, I forgot) to your daily routine. You can do it. Just start slowly and do it on a consistent basis. Consistency is the important factor.

Yes, you know that you will need to make a list of the changes that you may need to make in you present daily routine. You must list these activities so you can view them daily. This is your workbook, your guidebook, and I hope that you will use it to your advantage.

Now, list the steps that you intend to take below:

1. ______________________________

2. ______________________________

3. ______________________________

4. ______________________________

5. ______________________________

Why Isn't My Make-up Working?

Change is hard for all of us. If you have been using the same make-up techniques for the last ten years or more, it may well be time for a change. I would suggest you invest in several books and magazines that illustrate make-up application and the products that will help you to achieve the look you are striving for. Okay, you don't exactly know what you are striving for. We all feel that way from time to time. We have heard all the hype; don't wear more make-up as you grow older, don't wear light lipstick or you will look young and foolish (hey, maybe we like young and foolish), don't wear false eyelashes or you will look harsh, and don't line your lips with a dark liner because your lipstick will bleed... I could go on, but I am sure you get the picture. What you need to decide is what look you actually like. As you might do if you were redecorating your living room, collect pictures of make-up colors and styles that please you and put them with this workbook. You will soon see a trend and may be able to decide what look and colors please you. This is a good first step.

If you are like I am, you have worried for many years as to what colors are best for you. I have been a cool, and then a warm, and then back to a cool. Now, I tend to buy what I think looks best on me. We will talk more about that in the chapter on clothes. However, many make-up companies are embracing the warm and cool aspects of make-up, and that might be very helpful to you. You will need to experiment with different looks. Don't be afraid to try something new. If you have a daughter or a granddaughter, I am sure she would be happy to experiment on you. Try it.

I am not going to suggest any brands or companies. I will admit to trying everything from the very expensive that I bought in Paris to the least expensive that I found at a local discount drugstore. I am still looking for that perfect lipstick color or that perfect eye shadow. This is what you must do. If you have never enjoyed make-up or the application of it, you might make an appointment with a professional for a lesson and then adapt the new techniques to your daily routine. Just experiment. You may just come up with a great new look!

One of the most important things you can do for yourself is consistent skin care. I know you have heard all your life that you shouldn't go to bed in make-up; well, it is true, you should not. I don't care how bad your head hurts . . . wash your face and at least put on a good moisturizer before you lie down. It is very important. I have not always practiced a great skin care routine until recently, and I can promise you that I can see a great improvement in a short time. I am not going to tell you what brand to buy since there are so many good ones on the market. If you have a friend with beautiful skin, as I have, ask her what she uses; she will surely share her routine and then you can follow her lead.

After a good skin care program, your make-up should be easier to apply and look much smoother. If you have good skin underneath, you will surely look wonderful in whatever make-up you choose. This may be the place to tell you one of my skin care secrets. I believe in microdermabrasion. I have been having that process done for at least the last nine years, and it makes a difference. It does not take the place of a consistent skin care routine; that is not the purpose of the procedure. If you have not considered microdermabrasion, then you should investigate the salons or doctor's offices in your location. As I am sure you probably know already microdermabrasion removes the top layer of dead skin and promotes a clearer, fresher complexion. In addition to clearer, it produces a hairless complexion. Yes, hairless. If you will look in a magnifying mirror (if you don't have one, get one today), you will see the fine hairs on your face. Shocked? Well, why do you think men have the ability, or so it seems, to age more slowly than we do? They shave daily and remove that top layer of dead skin and voila! Smoother skin. Do I want you to shave daily? If I said yes, you probably wouldn't finish this book, but consider this: After you have had microdermabrasion (either professionally or one of the home kits), you might want to "touch-up" if you see a few stray hairs. That is all I am saying. It certainly does help your make-up to go on smoother. Did I forget to mention that this process does seem to reduce the appearance of fine lines and wrinkles? If you do this, you will be very pleased. I'll say no more.

Let's talk about eye make-up. I have discovered recently that I need a more pronounced eye make-up. I noticed in pictures that I looked washed-out with my present eye make-up, so I started to apply with a heavier hand, which produced eyes that showed. You might try it. Don't let anyone tell you what you need to do. Experiment for yourself.

As for lips, you have heard that you need color; you may or you may not. I think you may need whiter teeth to make your lipstick look better and brighter. If you haven't tried the new products on the market that whiten teeth, what are you waiting for? You will be so pleased with the results. Of course, your dentist has the equipment to make your teeth white in one application. Save your money and ask him. It is a worthy investment.

The most important beauty tool that you should possess is the eyelash curler. My granddaughter knew what to do with one when she was three. I hope you use one daily, or at least when you go out. One secret that will help your lashes to stay curled is to use your blow dryer to heat your curler *slightly* before you use it. What a difference it can make in opening up your eyes! If you don't have one, put it on the list you will make at the end of this chapter.

Now is the time to decide to take a step in the direction of a newer and fresher look. You might want to start with a new lipstick and work your way into a new skin care routine. Whatever you do, you will surely be pleased with your efforts. Make a list of the beauty products and services that you are interested in trying. I would love to see your new look. Send me a picture!

Your List:

1. ____

2. ____

3. ____

4. ____

5. ____

What Do I Do with My Hair?

If you are going out into the world today, you may evaluate your looks by the way your hair behaves or misbehaves. That is normal. What is the first thing you notice about another woman? More than likely, it is her hairstyle, or perhaps the color of her hair. When we describe someone, we usually start with a description of her hair. Enough said, we all understand the importance of being satisfied with our hair. That is usually easier said than done. You may be a very fortunate woman who has a wonderful haircut and can "wash and go." Most of us do not fall into that category. So, what are we less fortunate ones to do? Let's explore some possibilities.

Let's talk about style. Now I don't mean all the styles that you see on the fashion runways or the latest cut that you might witness in your favorite hair salon. I want to focus on you. Or better yet, I want you to focus on you. What do you like? What makes you feel desirable? Let's play the age game again. If you were thirty or even forty, what would you do with your hair?

Most of you would let it grow longer, but you have bought into the myth that short hair makes you look younger… well, maybe not. I have been doing some private research on hair lengths, and I have come to the scientific conclusion (well, maybe not *that* scientific) that hair that covers a certain place on a woman's neck will subtract years and not add them. Now I don't mean hair that falls below your shoulders, but hair that is a few inches longer than what you have now. If you don't believe me, why don't you try on a wig that is close to your present hairstyle but a few inches longer? When you do, I believe you will see a small transformation. I know you will like it.

If you really don't see that the longer style is for you, then try very short hair. This may work for you. Just don't have a hair style that is ordinary… longer or shorter should work for you.

Still not convinced? Then try hair that is all one length. I have worn my hair like that for years. I have been advised that I need to update. I have tried, but it doesn't work for me. Again, go try on a wig that is one length and see how it works for you. I have had the length of my hair changed from time to time, and I assure you that I get more compliments on my hair when it is longer than a "woman my age" should wear.

After you have decided on a new style or a new version of your old style, you should investigate the use of color. If you have been using a color that is close to your high school or college color, you should rethink your choices. If you have dark hair, it may need to be softened to a different shade of your original hair color. As we age, we do need to soften or lighten the hair around our faces. Again, go to the wig salon to help you with your hair color decision. I believe you need a change in color if you have been holding on to a certain dark color for years.

If your hair is grey or light blonde, you may need to be aware of the variation of shades in your hair. We do not need to have hair all the same shade. Natural hair has variation. There are many new products on the market that promise this natural look. Your hair stylist and colorist will be happy to work with you. It is always wise to know what you want before you visit the salon. Magazines are a good source of hairstyles and colors to help you make that decision. Just do it! You will be pleased, I am sure.

One of the most important steps that you can take after you have settled on your style and color is the care that you will give your hair. I cannot impress on you enough what a regular conditioning program (the operative word being regular) can do for your style and color. There are so many good conditioners on the market that you can hardly make a bad choice. As I said, you must do this conditioning at least once a week. This is deep conditioning, not your daily rinse-out conditioner. When I do my deep weekly conditioning, I would scare anyone who came to my door. I rinse my hair and apply a generous amount of my conditioner. I then wrap aluminum foil around my head and place a shower cap over that. I wear this apparatus for several hours during which I use my hair dryer several times to heat the foil. Get the picture? If that is not bad enough, I usually have my teeth bleaching at the same time. Well, a girl has to do maintenance.

You know what you must do. Make your plans for your hair makeover, if that is what you need. There is something about making a list that helps you get these tasks done. So, do it now, list what you plan to do. Go for it!

Your List:

1. ____________________

2. ____________________

3. ____________________

4. ____________________

5. ____________________

Why Do I Have Nothing to Wear?

This is the most difficult chapter for me to write. I am glad you cannot peer into the inner sanctuary that I call a closet. My friends are not allowed inside the door of this room, and I know they are getting very tired of hearing me confess that I am going to "work on it soon." I am afraid to throw anything away for fear that I might just lose the last five pounds and be able to wear the garment. I am sure you understand. Nevertheless, no one needs fifteen pairs of jeans in various styles and especially sizes. I must do something! Does your closet resemble this description? If you are a neat, organized, *I know where everything is* girl, then go on to the next chapter and leave this one to those of us who need it.

This is the first step I think we should take . . . get a cup of coffee and then decide how much time you want to spend on this project. If you are not totally dissatisfied with your closet and arrangement of your clothes and accessories, then you may not need to spend the time on this project. If you are, then let's go. First, do not take everything out of the closet. If you do, you will have an overwhelming pile of clothes that you may want to throw away before you even sort. I know what the books say; I have tried this, and I don't recommend this to anyone over fifty. This just takes too long, and we have better things to do!

Start with small steps. Spend ten or fifteen minutes just straightening the shelves and hangers. Don't discard anything, just make everything look neater. Pick the shoes up off the floor and put them in boxes or hang them on shoe racks. If you knew me well, you would know that I have many, many, many shoes that I do not wear. They are so beautiful that I cannot bring myself to throw them away. I will never wear them because they hurt, but that is not the point. We all have our little secrets. Mine just happens to be shoes.

Now that you have neatened the room, start hanging the same colors together, and you will see that you have fifteen white shirts and possibly wear only two. I won't tell you to throw away anything, but at least you will know what you have. After you have hung the colors together, you will see a pattern in your choice of colors and fabrics. At this point you should have everything of the same color together. Go through the different colors and decide what you like and don't like. If it looks good on you, then leave it hanging. If it doesn't, take it out and place it in a box to store. I am not going to tell you to throw it away or give it away; you are not ready to give up any of these precious family members. I understand how you feel, since I have clothes older than my grandchildren. Now that you have carefully put away these closet stuffers, go back into the closet and rearrange the pieces that you have left. At this point you should hang the blouses together, skirts together, and pants together. You get the picture. I know it looks better.

Look at your shoes now. How many pairs do you actually wear? I thought so. Do the same for the shoes. Don't throw or give them away, just put them in storage and get them out of the closet. Your thoughts may be turning to purses now. I really don't think you have to do the same for purses. Just straighten them and you may find a treasure that you have forgotten.

By this point your closet is really taking shape. You have the clothes that you wear most in order and can start deciding the pieces that you may need to add to make your wardrobe more workable. This is the hard part. Have you ever wondered why you spend a fortune on a dress or suit that you may wear only once or twice for a special occasion and have to spend less on clothes that you wear on a daily basis? As I have grown older, I have decided that the bulk of my clothing budget should be spent on the clothes that I wear the most. Don't spend a week's pay on a pair of heels that hurt when you could spend that amount on a pair of great loafers that you might wear almost daily and feel great in each time. I do that, and it works.

As you are pondering over the pieces to buy to make your wardrobe more workable, you should think quality over quantity. You probably need better clothes, not more clothes. As we age, we need to be keenly aware of fit, and it is hard to get a good fit in an inexpensive garment. It is better to have one well-fitting jacket than a closet full of misfits. As we age, we need to think simplicity in dressing. Take off that necklace, it is probably too much. Wear a simple, but well-tailored white blouse (or off-white) and a pair of well-tailored black pants to which you may add a black vest to keep the line clean and see what it does for you. Solid colors seem to look more elegant than prints. Someone advised me when I was a young woman on a very tight budget to buy black in a size larger than I thought I needed to look like a well-dressed lady. That has always stayed with me, and I still think it is good advice.

I know you are wondering about the clothes you have carefully packed away. I suggest you put them in storage for now and forget them. You will want to revisit these garments in the distant future and search for hidden treasures. If no treasures are found, you may want to donate the entire container to a charity or take the best pieces to a consignment shop and invest the profit into a new garment.

I have always been a shopper. I could even be considered very good at what I do; or, so I thought. I have a lot of clothes. I am not in love with many of them. I buy most of my clothes on sale. I can walk into a store and, as if by radar, go to the best sales, which may be my biggest mistake. I have closets full of lovely sale items. You have done the same thing. How could I have not bought the expensive blouse when it was marked down to twenty dollars? Have you ever wondered *why* it was still on the rack? Evidently, it wasn't selected to go home with anyone else. Of course, I am not saying that you cannot find a great bargain that you will love and will be a great addition to your present wardrobe; I am saying to make that selection very carefully. My best shopping advice when adding to your new and organized closet is to absolutely love the garment you are buying. Don't put it on and ask your friend or the salesclerk if it looks good on you. If you don't put it on and absolutely love it in the privacy of your dressing room do not take it home with you. It will become one of the storage items during your next closet makeover. So, love it or don't buy it; enough said?

Since you feel energized over your closet makeover, let's talk about foundations... isn't that an old-fashioned word? Actually, foundation is a very appropriate term to use in reference to the garments that you should wear under these new or recycled garments. How long has it been since you were measured for a new bra? According to research, most women wear the wrong size. Buying a bra is like buying blue jeans; the process is certainly harrowing, but when you find the right one, the result is priceless. In the correct fitting bra you will look younger and thinner. If that is not enough to get you to the closest department store, then nothing else will do it. After you have found the perfect bra (I know *perfect* is a strong word, but some new bras are close to it), you should look for new panties. If you will try on the ones with high-cut legs, you will be surprised as to the length you will add to yours. You may also investigate the pant-liners that give you a smooth line from waist to toe. Just look, what have you got to lose but the look of a few extra pounds? After you have armed yourself with a new arsenal of attractive and well-fitting undergarments, go home and enjoy the difference in the way your clothes fit. You will see that your bosom is lifted and your stomach is flatter… Now, how nice is that?

Now we are to the part that you have to write something. I have been doing all the talking and suggesting in this chapter on clothes, closets, and undergarments. I know that you surely have decided to make some changes; so, list them in the space below and get busy!

I will:

1. ______________________________

2. ______________________________

3. ______________________________

4. ______________________________

5. ______________________________

Why Isn't My House What I Want?

If you are completely satisfied with your home, then go on to the next chapter, give the book away, or read this chapter anyway and try to understand what the rest of us are going through. Most of us vacillate between walking into our homes, especially after a trip, and thinking how wonderful everything looks to wanting to rearrange everything including the husband and the dog and probably in that order. Of course, we have all visited a friend who has a beautiful home, has a demanding job (still!), and cooks for the homeless. I don't cook for the homeless or anyone else. However, after such a visit, I return home just a little dissatisfied with the way everything looks. I want to do something; I don't know what. My decorating looks dated, not fresh enough. You may have had the same experience.

If you want to do some minor changes that will give you a fresh look, or at least make you more satisfied and comfortable in your home, think large. I don't mean a large bill at your favorite furniture or design store, but large in the new accessories you might buy to change the look of your rooms. Most of us have had enough years to gather all the treasures that we could never part with and must leave sitting on all of the available space in our already crowded rooms. So, gather these treasures and either make them a collection (putting them together in one place), or carefully store them away for an extended period of time. Remember the treasures from your closet, do the same with these treasures. Now, with the new spaces you are ready to decorate with a new eye.

As you look around these spaces that are devoid of "things," picture a large (yes, very large) vase or container in that space. Not only will you have a new and exciting focal point in your room, you will have visually added more space. As you begin to search for these new and large accessories you may find, as I did, that large and impressive accessories are pricey. You can do as I did. Look around junk stores or garage sales and find the ugliest large vase or container that is a color no one would dare put into a beautiful room and make an offer on it. You will probably be able to buy this treasure for a mere penance or possibly be paid to remove it from the premises. No one would believe that this will become one of the focal points in your new decorating scheme. After you have gotten this ugly creation home, you should hide it in the garage for the next few days as you buy the spray paint to transform it into a work of art. Yes, spray paint should do it. I have covered several large, ugly pottery pieces with spray paint and found a place for them that surprised even me. I used white paint, which does an amazing transformation, but feel free to use the color that best supports your color scheme. Place the piece in a strategic spot and get ready to be praised for your decorating skills.

Now that you have made these changes, you may be ready for a few more. I have found that lamps are an easy and inexpensive way to update. Look around your rooms. Wouldn't you like to remove the lamp that you bought when you married? We do not throw any valuable treasure away; we just place it in a storage spot and worry about it later. At least you will have everything in a storage bin for a garage sale or donation. There is something about not throwing away my valuable, but useless, items which lessens the guilt of buying new. You may have a different method. Let me know. I might like your method better. Nevertheless, this works for me.

If you have removed the small "set-arounds" (I have a friend who calls all the items his wife buys "set-arounds," and I think that is a great term for all the items that get clustered on our tables and shelves) and have replaced them with large and bold accessories, and you have replaced your lamps, then you are seeing a wonderful transformation. You may want to do one more important change. Look at your window treatments. You might want to consider two options The first look that you might investigate is wooden blinds, or, should I say, the look of wooden blinds. I replaced my living and dining room blinds for the look of wooden blinds for a ridiculously low price. No one knows it because the new plastic blinds have the look of real wood. Just be sure you measure carefully or have a professional do it for you. It is well worth the effort for this great new look. I know, I did say two options. The second option is sheers that puddle on the floor falling from rods that are attached an inch from the ceiling. It is a great look for a fraction of the price of custom-made drapes. I used black wrought iron rods and off-white sheers. The look is dramatic.

I know I said the window treatments would be the last important change, well, I was wrong. You need to look at your floors. I believe in rugs. I love rugs. Rugs cover a multitude of sins. You may be thinking that you need new carpet, and you might, but I strongly believe that money could be invested in a wonderful rug that you would have in any place that you might move in the future. I don't mean little throw rugs; I mean large, luxurious rugs that make a fashion statement. I can hear you thinking that you may not be able to afford these rugs... You are wrong. Buy the best solid color shag rug that you can find and buy its twin at the same time and put them together with duct or rug tape and voila! A great rug that will make any room elegant.

When you complete any of these projects, you will see your home in a new and refreshing light. It sometimes takes small changes to make us satisfied or even thrilled with what we have. As I age, I find that it really does take very little to make me happy. My problem is getting started on the project. Just do it! As you know, it is time to make your list. I suggest that you go into each room and decide what you could do to add new life to the space. So, list below what your plans are:

I want to:

1. ______________________________

2. ______________________________

3. ______________________________

4. ______________________________

5. ______________________________

Why Do I Worry about Everything?

I am a professional worrier. I believe that I have a genetic flaw in my personality. I understand that my grandmother was also a professional worrier. Consequently, I inherited her talent for projection worrying. I will explain. Projection worrying is being anxious about situations that, in all probability, will never happen. For example, I can worry about the condition of the traffic on the interstate during a trip that I am planning to take three weeks from now. I can imagine that it might rain, or even worse "ice," during that fifteen minutes that I might be on the highway. If you have ever done that, then you understand; if not, skip the next example. When my grandson was born, my daughter was worried that his bride's parents (he was three hours old) would not give him the proper rehearsal dinner. I had to reassure her that I would handle the occasion. I completely understood her worry even though I didn't think it compared to my worry, which I can't exactly remember now. It was important at the time.

On a more serious note, we all have a Biblical mandate to take care of our families. We believe that we are required as women to worry about our children's welfare. Yes, we are to be concerned and mindful of our children's spiritual, physical, and emotional states. If we have, at their birth, dedicated them to the Lord, then we should try and leave our concerns and worries with Him for their lifetimes. Does that not work for you? It should, but in our human condition most of us have a hard time with this very simple act. Why is it so hard for us to leave the care of our children in the hands of the creator of the universe? Or why do we believe that we have entrusted their care to Him, but find ourselves taking back something we need to worry about? When you find yourself in this condition, think of the sparrow. I was enmeshed one day in a serious worry session (I can't remember the focus) when a verse that I had never noticed leapt from the pages of my Bible. The verse was Matthew 10:29 (NIV). I was very familiar with the verses of this much quoted passage, but I had failed to focus on the promise that not one of these little birds will fall to the ground apart from the will of *our* Father. I just stopped and thanked the Lord for His care and rejoiced that we are more important than the little brown sparrow. I visited my daughter very soon after that and I noticed a new picture that she had just bought. It was, of all things, a little brown sparrow sitting on a piece of wood. She had bought a copy for me that I have in my dressing room so I can look at it as I dress every morning. Isn't God good?

Well, you are thinking that this is all good advice, but that I don't have a clue of all the things that you have to worry about. Maybe I do. Remember, I am sixty-two, and have been divorced, broke, widowed, upset, confused, and tired. I have gone through all the "if-only-I-had" scenarios that you can possibly imagine. You have to stop. You have to focus on the things that you can accomplish now with God's help and step out in faith. He can use you. You don't have to be anything but willing, and He has a very special place for you to serve. The very best part about serving is that you may not have time to worry.

You may still not be convinced that you can give up the worry habit. I understand since I have been dealing with this particular bad habit all my life. Remember, I am not a psychologist (I have a dear friend who is. . . . Does that count?), but I do believe that we must replace the negative thoughts in our consciousness with the calming and peaceful thoughts that we should embrace. When you start to worry, quickly replace that thought with a mundane thought, and you will immediately feel a sense of relief. Try it. For example, if you are worrying about your child (I know they never grow up, but that is for another book), you need to think of how you want to rearrange your closet or the new purse that you may buy. Understand? Think of anything to get your mind focused on another subject. It sounds simple, but it seems to work.

We are now going to embrace a very serious subject that might be the real basis for your worry. Are you afraid to die? I know you may be upset with me since this has been a fun book and now I am talking about the one subject most people avoid, and that is death. The next statement is the most important statement in the book: *Until you are not afraid to die, you can never really live.* To not be afraid to die you must have a relationship with Jesus Christ. It is very simple... faith in Christ. You then belong to Him, and you can live the rest of your life knowing your destiny. If you will notice, I said you *can*, I didn't say you *would.* As Christians, we sometimes forget who we belong to and where we are destined. I have done that many times. I used to be afraid to fly. I would worry that the plane would crash, be hijacked, or bombed. One day I realized that God has a plan for me, as He does for you, and I was either going to arrive in Dallas to see my daughter and her family or heaven to see Jesus, and I was excited about either place.

This final and what I consider the most important chapter of this book is not unlike the preceding chapters because I will ask you to take an active part in eliminating some of your worries and worry activities. I want you to make a list of the major worries that you had ten years ago. Hard to do, isn't it? Unless you had a devastating illness in your family, serious financial problems, or emotional problems, you will more than likely not be able to recall these situations. What about six months ago? I thought so. Then let's look at the present. I know you can do that. List your five major worries with possible solutions and date them.

Now commit these worries to the Lord and ask for His guidance.

1.____

2.____

3.____

4.____

5.____

Now fold the page or put a piece of paper over what you have written. I want you to revisit this page in thirty days and see what God has done for you because, remember, you are worth more than many sparrows (Matthew 10:31).

Epilogue

Thank you for reading this book and going on this journey with me. Aging is indeed a fascinating experience, and I feel as if I have talked to a friend as I have shared my thoughts with you. I hope that you will keep this book and indeed use it as a guide and handbook to chart your progress in the years to come. You may be the friend who will have great ideas for our next book, which could be... *Seventy is Sizzling!* My prayers are with you and may you be excited with your life as you learn to say... *Sixty... So What?*

In His Love,

Sharon